Para-What?

SARA ROCKFORD

PAGE PUBLISHING, INC.
New York, NY

First originally published by Page Publishing, Inc. 2019

ISBN 978-1-64584-159-3 (Paperback)
ISBN 978-1-64584-160-9 (Digital)

Printed in the United States of America

Disclaimer

To my Rockford Mass Transit District Paratransit Drivers, honestly, you guys are the best. It really takes a special kind of person to do the type of work that you do on a daily basis. I salute you, or should I say that, I salute a nice chunk of you, for your hard work and your devotion as well as your dedication to your chosen profession.

You really have to be a people person, dealing with a whole lot of different personalities, some of which, it is sad to say, are dwelling in one single body. This statement encompasses not only the passengers but your fellow coworkers as well. I have been on those little vans where I have heard drivers talking to themselves. It is kind of scary stuff for them to be behind the wheel of what could be deemed a deadly weapon and holding full-blown conversations with themselves. However, for those of you keeping it real and performing the job from your heart, my hat goes off to you.

I truly believe that you work hard at what you do, and at times, I know for a fact that you go severely unnoticed, unrecognized, and unappreciated. There are a few of you out there who I actually love, and it is rare that you don't cross my mind at least once or twice a day.

There are those of you who I would actually like to hang out with outside of the world of paratransit. You seem as if you would be just so cool to hang out with and just talk about whatever crosses the mind. Then there are those of you, well I will just leave it at that, because such uses of extreme colorful vocabulary are simply not ladylike. I believe one of my favorite cartoon characters refers to those colorful vocabulary words as "sentence enhancers." Again, I shall not be using such language to describe you. But know that all of you are in my prayers.

Well, to be honest once again, the bulk of you are in my prayers. Oh, please forgive me and allow me to take what I just said back. You all are in my thoughts and prayers. It is just some of you get that extra five minutes of prayer time because I really like you.

I have heard a few things over the years during my times riding paratransit that I figured would make a good comical book. I figured, what the hey, if not me, then someone else probably would have done it if it hasn't already been done.

All the short stories listed in this book are extreme exaggerations with a little touch of the truth. Some of them I have heard from the drivers, some from passengers, and even some I have experienced for myself. All names have been changed and identities have been altered to protect the innocent as well as the guilty. I'll leave it up to you to decide which passenger, driver, and or even office personnel are in the hot seat for a particular story. But don't rack your brains too hard because the character or characters and maybe the entire story could be totally and unequivocally fake. Ha, I'll never tell.

I sincerely hope that you will find this book funny and be able to laugh. Proverbs 17:22 states, "A merry heart doeth good as a medicine: but a broken spirit drieth the house." The last time I checked the dictionary, *merry* means to be very happy, cheerful, to have a feeling of joy and happiness.

This is one of my goals, that you will be merry after reading this book. I seriously hope that you will not become offended and try to hunt me down with torches and pitch forks. Well, let me bring it into today's times. I hope you will not hunt me down with forty-fives and automatic machine guns. I bruise easily. But just in case you do, I am using a pseudonym. Until someone blesses me with a gazillion dollars, I still have to utilize your services, and I would rather be safe than sorry. Who knows, maybe writing this book will make me a gazillionaire. Even if that did happen, I would still ride paratransit because I consider quite a few of you as my friends. Not to mention, I have indeed met some really great people who also utilize the RMTD paratransit service. So please sit back and enjoy the many adventures of Para-What?

Regards,
Sarah Rockford

Contents

My Sandwich 9

May I Schedule a Ride, Please? 16

Paratransit Survival Kit...21

I Believe I'm Being Stalked! 26

You're a Stinking Liar 34

Look Out Fixed Route 45

Paratransit Newbies..50

Compassion 57

The Hated Driver..64

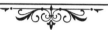

My Sandwich

It is indeed a wonderful blessing and an honor to grow up in a family where creativity and God-given talent flows throughout the majority of the gene pool. Although not publicly famous, we have singers, songwriters, artists, and we even have carpenters.

When we were younger, my little sister who had an extremely amazing voice, created a catchy little ditty, and she named it *My Sandwich*. Although I seriously doubt that it would have made Billboard's Top 100 List, it was an adorable and catchy little tune nonetheless. In her song, she sang about the description of a sandwich, which in glowing terms was simply "No good." She listed a number of reasons why this poor little sandwich didn't come up to code. For starters, there was way too much mayonnaise. All that rich, white, creamy, gooey stuff oozed out the sides of the bread.

Another reason why this sandwich failed to be appealing was because of the cheese, which was covered in disgusting mold. Finally, the last downfall to this sandwich were the elusive pickles that somehow kept falling out of the dang thing. The mystery still remains to this day behind how the pickles managed to escape from the sandwich, and it's probably one mystery that will never get solved.

Even though thinking about my sister's song brought back wonderful childhood memories and even made me wonder why anyone in the world would write a song about a disgusting sandwich, there is a current and even better sandwich of whose story that I would like to share.

Julie stepped onto the steps of the paratransit van, tiredly elated that it finally showed up. She had clocked out over an hour ago, and that's how long it took for the van to finally make its grand appearance outside her work. She was whipped, frustrated, and desperately needed to go straight home. It had been an emotionally and physically taxing day for her.

Everyone and their mother, it seemed, wanted or needed her to perform personal tasks that were all declared important. She heard her name called so many times that she honestly didn't know whether or not she was coming or going. Her head was literally spinning. Not only did she have to deal with the demands of her superiors but she also had to deal with the pain of her two prosthetic legs that were in dire need of replacement.

Honestly, they had long since served their purpose. They were scratched, banged up, beat up, and in some places, chipped. Where she attached the prosthetics to her partial limbs, they pinched her something fierce. The fifty extra pounds she had lovingly acquired didn't quite help the situation either. But nevertheless, she somehow managed to always meet the demands of her superiors and sometimes going beyond what they expected of her. She refused to let her disability get the better of her.

Julie was familiar with the driver who showed up to take her home. His name was Greg Edmonds. She liked him well enough, but she didn't care that he pulled up today in one of the older and clunkier paratransit vans. The seats were bunched together like sardines in a can, and the seatbelts were often very difficult to fasten around her slightly expanded waistline. Maneuvering around in this compressed fiberglass can on wheels was difficult to say the least. It even contributed to some of the damage done to her prosthetic legs.

This van was so horrible that Julie took it upon herself to call in to the office to see if something could be done about it—replace it, retire it, sell it. It didn't matter just as long as it was pulled out of service. Apparently, as she slowly stepped onto the van, her prior written and verbal concerns, complaints, and griefs fell on deaf ears because the clunky van was still in service, still being utilized to pick up passengers.

The paratransit driver, Greg, for the most part, was kind enough and sort of okay on the eyes. In Julie's opinion, he wasn't a perfect ten, maybe a three or a four. However, Greg carried himself as if he was truly the perfect gift to all women. How he managed to think that about himself was beyond Julie's comprehension and imagination.

He had a full head of curly hair, and there was a big splash of gray hair in the middle of his head that ran from front to back. The part of his hair that wasn't gray was a deep, rich, black color, almost blue-black in appearance. Julie often wondered whether or not Greg dyed his hair but hoped that this creation was a freak of nature and not something that was done on purpose.

Julie's personal and private nickname for him was skunky, but she dared not share this information with any of the other paratransit riders and or any of the other drivers for fear of it leaking out. She didn't want Greg to find out that he was privately nicknamed for an ugly, stinky, pee-spraying rodent.

On occasion, when Greg pulled up in front of Julie's work, he would be rather cranky. Although to Julie's knowledge, he never took his frustration out on any of the passengers, nor did he on her. However, it definitely came out in the way that he drove and handled the van. On those days when Julie's path crossed Greg's, and he was in one of his moods, she knew to avoid eye contact, find a seat, buckle up, and hold on for dear life. Posted speed limits were a blur, pedestrians became moving targets, and if a passenger stepped on the van with a full stomach, it wouldn't stay full for long.

On this particular night, Greg was in a wonderful mood, which surprised not only Julie but the other two passengers that were already seated on the van. Even though Greg was driving the van from hell, Julie was taken aback at how friendly and cordial Greg was toward her.

"Hi, beautiful," he said to her, which was something that he had never said before.

"Oh my, you look as if you had a horrible day today."

Shocked at this kind outburst of intuition, Julie could only nod her head in agreement.

"Step on up, my dear," Greg said to her, waving her into the van.

"Please find yourself a seat and make sure that you buckle up. I will try my best to get my sweet angel home right away."

"Okay," Julie managed to say, stepping deeper into the van. She acknowledged the other two passengers and found a seat and buckled up as instructed.

As the driver made his rounds dropping off the other passengers at their respective homes, he turned around to Julie and said, "I have saved the best for last." Julie smiled in kind, still in shock at how nice and cordial Greg was to her.

"Julie," Greg said softly while waiting for a traffic light to turn green, "I hope you don't mind, but I need to make a stop before I drop you off. You are my last passenger for the day, and I will not have any time to do what I need to do after I get off work today."

Julie looked at him and pondered for a moment over this strange request and finally said, "Sure, I guess it would be okay." But honestly, Julie really didn't care how much time Greg did or didn't have after getting off his job. She just wanted to go home and crash.

"Oh, thank you," Greg said, slapping his hands together before turning around to take hold of the steering wheel again.

"You are a real doll!"

Five minutes later, they pulled in front of a small convenience store where Greg unbuckled his seatbelt and quickly hopped out of the van. Before shutting the door, he yelled back at Julie over his shoulder, "This will only take a few seconds, sweetie!" Before Julie could acknowledge him, Greg made a mad dash into the store.

Fifty minutes later, he emerged from the store carrying four grocery bags full to capacity. Julie looked at him and sighed heavily as she watched him approach the van.

"Some whole dang fifty minutes of my life just gone, poof, and for what," Julie quietly mumbled to herself.

"Oh, thank you so much, my dear. I really appreciate you making this sacrifice for me," Greg said upon returning to the driver's seat.

"You have saved me so much time. Now, my sweet dear, I can finally take you home."

"Huh, Skunky, you are so not even welcome," Julie said under her breath rather hotly.

Another fifteen minutes had passed before Greg pulled the paratransit van in front of Julie's house. Julie sighed heavily and unbuckled herself from the seat. As she gathered up her things, she noticed Greg was fishing around in one of his grocery bags looking for something. As to what that something was, Julie really didn't care. All she knew was that she desperately wanted to get off the van and get into her house.

As Julie approached the front of the van to exit, Greg handed her what looked like a sub sandwich. It was wrapped in clear plastic with a huge label affixed to it describing it as a cold-cut combo with lettuce, cheese, salami, turkey, and ham.

"Now, sweetheart," Greg said, smiling up at her from the driver's seat, "you got a microwave, right?"

Julie said yes without really thinking twice about the question. "Now, this here sandwich tastes really good if you stick it in the microwave and warm it up for about forty-five seconds." Shocked at this kind gesture, Julie took the sandwich, smiled at the driver and said, "Thank you," before exiting the vehicle.

Wasn't that a nice thing for Greg to do? she thought to herself upon entering her house and dropping her purse and other belongings just inside the door. *I guess he was feeling sorry and wanted to make up for taking the fifty minutes he stole from my life, and now I don't even have to cook dinner tonight.*

"Hallelujah!" Julie shouted in excitement. This day wasn't so bad after all.

Julie removed the sandwich's wrapping paper, placed it on a plate, and put it into her microwave. She set the timer for exactly forty-five seconds and went to her refrigerator to grab a can of grape soda. As the microwave beeped, alerting Julie that it was time to remove the sandwich, she grabbed a couple of napkins that rested on her kitchen counter top and retrieved the sandwich from the microwave. She walked over to her kitchen table and placed her meal on the table. After plopping down into one of her kitchen chairs, she lowered her head, closed her eyes, and said a quick prayer of thanks before she began to eat.

The sandwich looked and smelled heavenly. Julie opened her soda and heard the soft, fizzy sound of the acid in the pop and raised it up to her mouth to take a quick sip before she tore into the sandwich. She sat the soda down on the table and then wrapped her hands around the sub and began to bring it to her mouth. Her mouth watered in anticipation of the first bite.

All of a sudden, she heard a loud banging on her front door.

"Who in the world could that be?" she said aloud. As she returned the sandwich to the plate, she rose and walked over to her door to see who was interrupting her free meal.

"Who is it?" Julie politely said, somewhat cautious of the voice on the other side of the door.

"Have you warmed up my sandwich yet?" the voice shouted back from the other side of the door.

"What the what!" Julie heard herself scream out.

"I said, is my sandwich ready?" the voice yelled once again.

"Give me a second," Julie said without opening her door.

"Really! I can't believe the nerve of some people!" she blurted out as she returned to the kitchen and gathered up the sandwich, feeling rather lucky that she hadn't tossed the wrapping paper into the trash. She carefully re-wrapped the sub, still in heated disbelief.

"I can't believe this crap."

Julie opened her front door to see the paratransit driver, Greg, standing at her front door with a slight look of anger on his face.

"Gees," he said as Julie handed him the sandwich and continued rather heatedly, "that was clearly more than forty-five seconds. I hope you haven't destroyed my sandwich by adding anything extra to it."

"No," Julie said, shaking her head somberly, still in disbelief.

Without saying a single word of thanks, Greg took the sandwich, turned, and headed back to the idling paratransit van. Julie stood there watching him as he climbed into the driver's seat, shut the door, unwrapped his sandwich, and began to devour the thing.

She watched as he pulled what looked like a bottle of soda from one of his bags, uncapped it, and took a deep drag from the bottle.

Greg finished the sandwich in under seven minutes, topped off his soda, and pulled away into the darkness. It took Julie another five minutes for her to gather herself together before retreating into the comfort of her now sandwich-less home.

Please let this be a lesson to you who receive things from the drivers. You must be a thousand percent sure that what they are giving you is really what they are giving you with no take backs. Because if you don't, you will end up sandwich-less as well as still hungry, exactly like our dear Julie. And might I add, totally ticked off.

May I Schedule a Ride, Please?

Amanda picked up her phone to place a call in to the paratransit office to schedule herself a round-trip ride. She had a routine doctor's appointment scheduled for this coming Friday and decided to call in a couple of days early to book the ride.

She sighed heavily as she punched in the numbers and waited for the call to be connected. As usual, instead of a live person picking up, she was greeted with the normal recorded message.

"Welcome to the Rockford Mass Transit District. To better serve you, all calls may be recorded. For routes and schedule information please, press one. For paratransit services please, press two." Amanda gently pushed the number two button on her keypad and waited for the next recorded voice.

"Thank you for calling the Rockford Paratransit office. All calls may be recorded. If you need a ride, please hold and the next operator will help you. If you are calling after 6:30 p.m., please hang up and dial 8-1-5-9-6-1-2-2-5-0." Amanda waited patiently while the recorded messages droned on.

"Please hold while I try that extension," the recorded voice said. For a brief moment, Amanda thought she hit the jackpot and became excited at the prospect of talking to someone right away, but then, the next recorded voice started to speak, and Amanda's quick shot of excitement was soon abated.

"Thank you for calling. Please hold, and your call will be answered as quickly as possible," the familiar message voice said. *All lies,* Amanda thought to herself as she waited to talk to a living and breathing individual. But then again, she knew deep down in her soul that this was the norm of scheduling a ride on paratransit. Why she thought she would be connected right away was beyond her. Sometimes wishful thinking is just a waste of valuable energy.

"Thank you for calling Paratransit, this is Peaches," the voice on the other end finally said after Amanda spent a long ten minutes' worth of listening to uneasy easy listening music.

"How may I assist you today?"

"Peaches!" Amanda exclaimed somewhat loudly without thinking.

"Did you say that your name was Peaches?"

"Yes, ma'am," the young lady responded back in kind.

Oh my, Amanda thought to herself, *How in the world could someone name their precious little baby after a piece of fruit?* Somehow sensing Amanda's thoughts, "Yes, I know my name is kind of on the weird side. But that was my mom's favorite fruit at the time she was pregnant with me and actually," Peaches continued, "I have a birthmark shaped exactly like a peach, in size and in color on the inner thigh of my right leg."

Shocked at this unsolicited piece of personal information, Amanda cleared her throat.

"Well, um, you must be new," Amanda said in an attempt to try and shift the conversation in a different direction, "I never heard your voice before, and I don't recall ever speaking to anyone named Peaches before."

"Yes, ma'am, as a matter of fact, I am new," Peaches said proudly, "I started here about three weeks ago, and I am truly loving every minute of working here. How can I help you today, ma'am?" Peaches repeated her rehearsed line.

"Well, Peaches," Amanda said, "my name is Amanda Johnson, and I would like to schedule a ride for this coming Friday. I have a—" But before Amanda could finish her sentence, Peaches abruptly said hold please and quickly placed Amanda on hold and into an unwelcomed chasm of music.

"Oh, well," Amanda said, placing her phone on speaker and then placing it on the cushion beside her on the sofa. Instead of bumming herself out over the delay, she decided to pick up her knitting and do a little multitasking while she was on hold with Paratransit.

She was almost finished with making a new baby blanket for her very first grandchild. Her daughter and her son-in-law, who lived out of state, decided not to find out the sex of the child. But instead decided to wait and see what God was going to bless them with.

Amanda respected their decision and decided to make a neutral colored blanket that would fit either a baby boy or a baby girl. But deep down, she was praying for a little grandson and hoped that her daughter would name him after her dearly departed husband, Charles. Amanda began smiling at the thought of holding her new grandbaby as she began to knit a new row.

"Thank you for calling Paratransit. This is Peaches, how may I assist you today?"

"Yes, Peaches!" Amanda shouted out as she placed her knitting into her lap and picked up her phone.

"This is Amanda Johnson, and I was calling to schedule a ride for this Friday. I have a doctor's appointment scheduled for that day and I need your service to get me there," Amanda said, smiling, her thoughts still on her unborn grandchild.

"Yes, Ms. Sandra Johnston," Peaches said, "allow me to look you up in our system."

"No," Amanda said, taking her phone off speaker and placing it in its natural position, "I said that my name is Amanda Johnson."

"Oh, I am so sorry, ma'am," Peaches said, "give me one second. Ah, here we are, Ms. Johansen. Now what day did you say that you wanted to schedule a ride for?"

"Peaches," Amanda said, speaking with a little bit more force and bass in her voice but trying not to sound flustered, "my name is Amanda Johnson, dear, and I would like to schedule a ride for this coming Friday, August 21."

"I am so very sorry," Peaches said, "I have only been her for three weeks, and during that time, the company decided to upgrade the telephone system. Instead of handheld devices, they equipped us with earpieces, and sometimes, they are not as clear as a regular phone."

"Oh, I understand dear," Amanda said, sympathizing with the young lady.

"Before I retired," Amanda continued, "I worked at a call center, and we had those same gadgets, and I never did get used to those rascals. They were something else, I tell you." As Amanda continued her sharing about the annoying earpieces, she softly heard Peaches say, "Whatever," and was taken aback at this young lady's rude behavior.

However, Amanda refused to allow Peaches to get under her skin.

"Well, Peaches, as I said before, I would like to schedule a ride for this coming Friday, August 21. I would like to go to 698 Featherstone and would like to be there at nine thirty in the morning and be picked up to go back home at 11:30 a.m."

Amanda heard the light tapping sound of fingers hitting a keyboard, but then all of a sudden, there was complete silence over the line. There was nothing, not even the annoying music. Amanda removed the phone from next to her ear and began to look at it as if it was the guilty culprit behind her disconnected call. Seconds later, she began to hear the beep, beep, beep sound of a disconnected call.

"What in the world!" Amanda exclaimed rather loudly, "I know that that little girl didn't just hang up on me." Amanda took in a deep breath before reciting her mantra.

"Five, four, three, two, one, two, three, four, the stress that I now feel has to walk out of the door. Six, five, four, three, two, one, two, and three, I know sweet Jesus you are helping me."

Amanda repeated her self-proclaimed, stress-relieving mantra a couple of more times before going into an impromptu prayer.

"Dear Lord," Amanda began to pray openly and rather loudly, "all I wanted to do was just schedule a simple roundtrip ride to the doctor's office. That's really all I wanted to do. How difficult was that? I realize that something as simple and as small as this should not have me all in a fluster. However, I must confess that I am rather ticked off at this moment. And that little girl said she had only been there for three weeks. So I should be the better person and show her some mercy. But it says in your word, Lord, that it would be better for a person to tie a huge stone around their neck and be cast into the sea rather than mess with a child of God. And I definitely belong to you, sweet Jesus, so you have to come through for me. Yes, yes, hallelujah!" Amanda said clapping her hands together in excitement.

"Also, dear Lord, I do realize that although I am old and gray, I still have it within my members to completely wipe that little rude girl off the face of this Earth. But I also realize that vengeance belongs to you, and I should just shut my mouth and stop complaining. But again, Lord, all I wanted to do was schedule a ride to the doctor's office, nothing major. At least I don't think that was anything major to do. So, Lord, in my closing, I thank you for allowing me to vent. Please forgive me for blowing this way out of proportion. Please forgive me for wanting to rip that little girl's head off her shoulders. Please have mercy on that little runt that works for Paratransit. And finally, when I do call back into the office, please don't allow Peaches to pick up the phone. Give me someone with a little bit more years on the job so that I can actually schedule a ride to the doctor's office for this Friday. In your sweet name, Amen."

Paratransit Survival Kit

I am quite sure that we have all heard of and maybe even some of us have used the expression *"Better safe than sorry."* This simple four-letter phrase covers a multitude of various situations where taking the time to plan something out far outweighs the consequences of not doing any planning at all. I am also quite sure that we have all had those moments where we have slapped ourselves on the forehead and said, "If only."

Riding Paratransit is no different. Each and every ride has to be planned out. Not to mention, each and every rider needs a paratransit survival kit to make sure that their ride will be a successful one, or they will end up on the sorry side of safety. You may be wondering why in heavens name I need a paratransit survival kit just to ride on the little white buses. Well, believe me, you do and please do not argue with me. I have been riding and or using the RMTD Paratransit services for the past thirteen years, and I think that I may know a thing or three.

A paratransit survival kit is essential to your well-being, your safety, and not to mention, your overall sanity. Depending on what I list, some of the items may be a bit on the pricey side. But don't worry because it is better to be safe than to be sorry. The following are items which you will need to make up your own personal paratransit survival kit, just in case you were wondering what the devil a paratransit survival kit actually is. Well, here it goes.

Just like how your athletes require special shoes to help them in their desired sport, you will need special shoes to ride on the paratransit buses. You may be asking, "Well, why can't my current shoes that I already have work?" Well, that is a very good question. And here is the reason why. But before I go into my explanations, I will let you know that you will need shoes with a good rubber sole. Please try to stay away from shoes that do not have any type of grip at the bottom of them at all. Also, for the ladies, please try to avoid wearing high-heel shoes. As a matter of fact, any shoes with a heel on them. The color of the shoes is not important at all. I will leave that decision up to you so be wild, free, and colorful.

Now, the reason why you need a good pair of shoes with rubber grips for the soles is because it can be rather dangerous getting on the bus and then walking to your seat. I believe the floor lining on the buses is made of rubber, but it acts and feels like some type of vinyl. There are ridges in the floor lining down the center of the bus. However, it doesn't provide much traction.

A person can still easily fall while walking toward their seat. This situation even becomes more dangerous during those times where rain and/or snow is tracked onto the bus. You may be thinking that it is the driver's responsibility to wipe down the center aisles of their bus if it is covered with water and or snow. Well, ha, and double ha. Please tell me what driver takes the time to wipe down the center of their bus, and I will purchase you lunch and dinner. However, since I am writing this book anonymously, that may be a little difficult for you to cash in.

The next item can be considered optional; however, it has proven to be very beneficial to me in the past. I will leave this one up for you to decide whether or not to get it. Nevertheless, you may want to purchase and have on you at all times—some type of a personal radio, MP3 player, or an audiobook player. Why would I need something like that? You may be asking. Well, here is why.

Granted, I do not have the best singing voice in all the United States, but neither do some of the paratransit drivers. Nothing irritates me more than listening to someone who absolutely cannot sing. Honestly, it is like listening to a cat and a dog try to perform a duet. The worst-case scenario would be a billy goat and a baboon coming together to write a love song and hope to perform it on the Stellar Awards. It just ain't happening.

Now, please don't get me wrong, some of the paratransit drivers have beautiful singing voices. There is one young man, I will not name, who I can listen to him sing the alphabet song all day long. And I promise you, I would be swooning from Earth to heaven and back again. It makes my toes curl just thinking about it. Again, this item is completely and totally optional. However, it doesn't hurt to have some type of device to block the noise. But your ears may be stronger than mine and may enjoy the screeching sounds of someone singing in a key that is not even an actual musical key.

Item number three deals with the type of clothing you wear. Before you even start fussing, I am not asking you to purchase paratransit-sanctioned clothes because there is no such thing. All I am asking you is to be careful of the type of clothing that you wear while riding on the paratransit busses. This may seem kind of off-the-wall, but I am talking from experience.

I made the horrible mistake of wearing something silky smooth on one of my paratransit trips. I can only assume that the driver forgot that he had passengers on the back of the bus. He made a quick turn, and I slid from one side of the seat to the next and almost fell to the floor. But I thank the Lord for having on good shoes with a strong rubber grip that prevented me from crashing to the floor. That fall would have hurt, and the groceries that I remember having with me would have scattered all over the bus. Not only would I have been in pain but my precious money would have been wasted from the destroyed groceries because I am quite sure I would have landed on top of some of them. I guarantee you that that wouldn't have been a pretty sight!

I am also not asking you to go out and purchase a brand-new wardrobe. Although I think that would be a rather lovely thing to do, at least for me anyway. All I am asking is that when you plan your paratransit trips, wear clothing that grips to the seat, like clothes made from cotton. Cotton has been my friend throughout my paratransit journey, and I surely appreciate it.

However, if you do test the limits and wear something silky and or satiny, please make sure that the seat belt that you are required to use is "gut-sucking-in" tight. Now, I must admit that at the time of my near tumble, my seat belt wasn't quite as tight as it should have been. It was a lesson learned.

The final thing needed in your paratransit survival kit is something that you probably already carry on your person. I know that I carry a small bottle of it in my bag. This little precious liquid can be seen being used at restaurants before meals and public restrooms. Yes, and even before and after shaking someone's hand. Yes, that's right, you guessed it. This precious little item is hand sanitizer. You probably do not need me to go into the reasons why you need hand sanitizer for the paratransit bus, but I will share with you anyway because there may be some things you may not know.

Most people, I included in that number, after boarding the paratransit bus, head straight for that first seat on the left-hand side. It is that seat that is right next to the lift gate. I was even told by one of the paratransit drivers that everyone loves that particular seat. I haven't a clue why.

However, since everyone loves it, it is indeed the filthiest, well speaking in terms of germs. In a way, it is a pretty cool seat because you have things in front of you that you can grab and hold of for safety purposes. For example, when the driver is either making a left or a right turn, you can grab hold of a silver bar that is mounted from the ceiling of the bus to the floor and hang on for dear life and lean with the turns. So I guess that would be one reason why I love that seat as well as countless other riders.

Since I have admitted that I have grabbed onto that bar, I am rather sure you have done the same thing. Why the need for the hand sanitizer? That is a very good question, and I am so glad you asked. Well, the following are the reasons: the common cold, influenza, and bronchitis just to name a few of the contagious things you could pick up just from sitting in that favorite seat.

Thank the Lord that I have never picked up any type of sickness, and I sincerely hope that neither have you. However, we all run the risk of catching something. But with our trusty little bottle of hand sanitizer, we can cut down on the chances of bringing something home with us that we did not want. On a sidenote, I was once told by one of the paratransit drivers that one of their passengers that they picked up from dialysis died in that same favorite seat. I don't know what bus number it was, and neither did the driver tell me, but how creepy is that? Granted, hand sanitizer may not prevent death, but it does fight off germs.

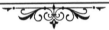

I Believe I'm Being Stalked!

"It's a good morning," Mandisa sang as Mable's alarm clock came to life. She had scheduled a ride on Paratransit the night before. She needed a few things for her household and decided to go to the Northridge Walmart on Alpine and Riverside. What she was going to Walmart for really was of no great significance. The things that she had on hand in her home probably would have sufficed. But the real reason behind her excursion was just so she could try her luck again at running into that hunk of a Paratransit driver named Curtis.

The time was now 7:00 a.m. And she knew she had to get up to get ready for her self-proclaimed man. She had been riding Paratransit now for the past seven days, hoping and praying that one of the drivers would be her Curtis. However, during those attempts she missed the mark every single time. She knew well enough that there was no guarantee that using the service would grant anyone the pleasure of riding with the driver they wanted to see and or ride with, or in her case, the driver of her lust filled dreams. Nor would it guarantee that they would have the same driver both going and coming.

One driver could easily take you to where you have to go, and a totally different driver could come back to pick you up and take you back home. Calling into the office to request a specific driver was a huge no-no and a colossal joke.

"These aren't your personal chauffeurs." She was told on several occasions when she did try to call the office to request Curtis specifically.

"Poo-poo on those office people," Mable said aloud while making her way to the bathroom, "and poo-poo on my seven-day stretch of bad luck. I am going to see my Curtis today come hell or high water."

As Mandisa beautifully sang, "It's A Good Morning," and Mable truly believed that it would indeed be a good morning.

"Hey 'C' Man," a fellow paratransit driver said while approaching Curtis, who sat comfortably in a break room chair, skimming over a newspaper. Curtis looked up from the paper and acknowledged the approaching man.

"What's up, bro?" Curtis said as he refolded the newspaper and placed it on the table for the next person to pick up and read.

"Hey, dude, I ran into your girl a couple of days ago," he continued while pulling up a chair.

"What girl?" Curtis said with a puzzled look on his face.

"Dude, stop playing. You know, the one," the young man said, starting to chuckle a bit, "she has been whole-heartedly stalking you for the last few years."

"Oh, you mean that one," Curtis said, sighing.

"Man, she has really got it in bad for you. All she did when she was on my bus was ask about you. 'Have you seen Curtis?' 'How is Curtis doing?' 'Is Curtis at work today?' 'Will you kiss Curtis for me?' 'Will you tell him that I want to have is love child?'" he said whimsically.

"You know, that lady of yours came really close to the edge of ticking me off and getting thrown off my bus," he now said with his voice becoming serious.

"Monty, cut her some slack, man," Curtis said, "she is probably just one of those lonely old ladies in need of some attention and companionship."

"Well, whatever it is," Monty said, rising from his seat, "I am so glad her heat-seeking, hormone-driven missiles are not pointed in my direction." Curtis smiled and shook his head as he rose to his feet.

"Come on," Monty said, waving his hand at Curtis, "it is now time for round two of the split shift."

"Just pray that I don't run into 'her' today," Curtis said as both men headed into the paratransit garage to retrieve their respective vehicles.

Mable sat in front of her vanity mirror. The counter top covered with beauty and antiaging creams, lotions, and scrubs. She had her tablet propped up near her on the counter with a YouTube video cued up on the proper way to apply foundation and how to create the smoky eye look. It had been a good little while since she used such things like eyeliner, lipstick, foundation, and mascara and was totally out of practice.

She was told by a dear friend that a person could easily find instructional videos on just about anything and everything on YouTube. Mable, being the driven person that she was, decided to check it out for herself, and she was in no way disappointed. She found exactly what she was looking for and then some.

As Mable sat there, looking at her reflection in the mirror, she wondered where had the time gone. She was still quite a looker, or so she had been told by the fellas at the Senior Center. A couple of them even asked her out for a date, but she refused them gracefully. The only person she was interested in was that sexy hunk of a paratransit driver named Curtis.

Mable's thoughts soon began to drift off, and she imagined Curtis standing behind her, gently brushing her hair. She imagined looking at him in the mirror, all six feet, two inches of him. Her eyes began to envision his broad shoulders, his muscular arms, and his elaborate chest that flowed to what Mable imagined to be the perfectly ripped stomach. His hands, although strong-looking, she imagined were soft and gentle to the touch.

It was clear that he was a mixture of two races, although Mable didn't know what two races they were. But he appeared to have inherited the best qualities of each. She figured that she would find that information out before she married him. A slight smile formed on Mabel's lips as her thoughts continued to drift, still imagining Curtis standing behind her.

Curtis had the most beautiful hazel eyes with thick luxurious eye lashes. He had a strong broad nose, not bulbous, but just big enough to handle all the kisses she would soon plant atop it. His lips were thick and full, and they were surrounded with a neatly cropped goatee that had little specs of gray throughout it. He had a strong and square jawline which Mable imagined tracing her fingers along while she cooed to him softly, and his voice was deep, rich, and velvety smooth like hot chocolate with marshmallows.

"This is zero eight five radio check," Curtis said, speaking into the radio's microphone, giving his van number to the dispatcher.

"Zero eight five, clear," a female voice responded back. As Curtis sat there in the van waiting for his turn to drive out of the garage, he scrolled down the van's tablet to see who would be his first pick up for the second half of his day. His face contorted a little when he saw that his first passenger would be Mable Kirkwood.

"Zero eight five to base," Curtis said, speaking into the microphone again.

"Zero eight five, go," the same female voice responded back.

"Um, can you, um," Curtis said, not totally able to make his thoughts turn into words.

"I don't understand. Um," the female voice said in response, laughing a bit.

"Base, never mind," Curtis said somberly, accepting his fate. He was going to try to ask if someone else could take Ms. Kirkwood but decided against it. *What harm could picking her up do?* he resolved within himself.

Twenty minutes later, Curtis pulled up in front of Mable Kirkwood's house. It was an adorable little house, almost picturesque. Everything seemed to have been in its place. The lawn was neatly mowed, and the hedges were nicely shaped. There was a small picket fence that ran around its perimeter, and there didn't appear to be a speck of debris in sight.

Curtis was actually impressed at the little home. Two minutes later, he saw the front door of the house opening and saw who he thought was Ms. Kirkwood emerging from the building. He did a double take as he saw a short, somewhat stout woman, slowly making her way down the walkway to the van. She was dressed in a black, way too tight, crushed velvet tracksuit, with a pair of Jordan's on her feet. What looked like a wig graced her head. It was brown in color with blond streaks, which cascaded down the sides of her arms and her back.

As Mable drew closer to the van, Curtis thought she must have been in some kind of a fight—which by the dark circles around her eyes, she had lost very badly. When she made it to the steps of the van, she looked up at him and smiled broadly, her bloodred lipstick staining her teeth.

"Hey, baby," Mable said, getting on the van, "it has been way too long since I have seen my sweetheart."

"I know," Curtis said, regaining his composure.

As Mable stepped up into the van, Curtis became overwhelmed with the overpowering scent of her perfume and quickly opened his driver-side window.

"So how have you been?" Curtis said, sucking in fresh air as Mable took the seat directly behind his.

"I've been better, but I am just fantastic now that I see you," she said, smiling from ear to ear.

"Oh, I'm no one special, ma'am," Curtis said in kind, "I'm just here to do my job."

The ride with Ms. Kirkwood wasn't actually too bad, Curtis thought to himself as he pulled up in front of the Northridge Walmart. But then again, he was doing fifteen miles over speed limit and tried his best not to engage in too deep of a conversation. He had driven so fast that he arrived at the store thirty minutes ahead of her scheduled drop-off time.

"Here we are, Ms. Kirkwood," Curtis said, opening the van's door.

"You take care now and try not to spend too much money," he said, trying to muster up a smile for her.

"Oh, you crazy, sexy thing, you," Ms. Kirkwood said, exiting the vehicle.

"If you come in with me I'll spend a little bit of money on you," Mable said, winking at him.

No thank you, ma'am, Curtis said mentally, rushing her off the van.

"I am really good. I don't need anything at the moment. Besides, it is against company policy for you to do that."

"Well, baby, I'll see you next time around," Ms. Kirkwood said, turning around to wave goodbye but not before placing her hands on her breasts, squeezing them and raising them up in a provocative manner. Curtis stared at her not knowing what to say and or do. Mable Kirkwood had completely taken him off guard. However, he was extremely grateful that she hadn't tried to kiss and or hug him this time around.

As Curtis sat idling in front of a passenger's house, waiting patiently for them to safely make it inside, he scrolled down the tablet to see what else he had for the day. His eyes popped when he saw that he had Ms. Mable Kirkwood on the return ride home.

"Dear Lord," he began to say, "I am so very sorry at whatever it was that I did to cause you to inflict this punishment upon me. I humbly ask, please let this cup pass." Curtis sat there in the idling van, drumming his fingers over the steering wheel, debating on whether or not to call into the office to see if Ms. Kirkwood could be pulled from his pickup list and inserted onto someone else's tablet.

That woman may try to kiss me this time, He horribly thought to himself. *And I don't want to have to physically hurt her or hurt her feelings by pushing her away.* Rather unexpectedly and all of a sudden, Curtis felt this sense of overwhelming peace cover him.

"Okay, Lord," Curtis said aloud as he put the van into gear and began to head toward Walmart and Ms. Kirkwood.

"Oh, blessed it be the name of the Lord," Ms. Kirkwood squealed as she saw that it was Curtis who had come back to pick her up. Curtis couldn't help but smile at the elderly woman as he saw her standing there clapping her hands in excitement.

"Why don't you just get on the van," Curtis said, "and I'll grab your bags for you and put them on the van. How does that sound, Ms. Kirkwood?"

"Oh, that would be just heavenly," she squealed in return.

"This normally doesn't happen to me," Ms. Kirkwood said, stepping onto the van and plopping down in the same seat she had earlier, "I rarely get to see the same driver on both trips, let alone my all-time favorite one."

"It is indeed rare, ma'am," Curtis said, placing the last grocery bag on the floor next to his passenger.

"I'm afraid I have one more pick up and drop off before I am able to take you home," Curtis said, returning to his seat and buckling up.

"Baby, that is okay," Ms. Kirkwood said excitedly, rocking back in forth in her seat, "you do what you gotta do. I am in no rush to get home. I have learned over the years not to buy anything that requires refrigeration if I have to use paratransit so nothing that I have is going to go bad."

Forty minutes later, Curtis pulled the paratransit van in front of Mable Kirkwood's home.

"Here we are," he said with a sigh of relief.

"Awe, poo-poo," Mable said, clearly getting upset that her time with Curtis was now coming to an end.

"I can take your grocery bags in if you like, ma'am. It won't be any trouble for me to do that for you."

Mable looked at him and smiled. "I would like that very much. You know, it amazes me," she continued, "that every time that I go into that dang store for one thing, I come out with that one thing and three other things besides it."

"It happens to me too," Curtis replied, smiling.

Curtis followed Mable into her home carrying her grocery bags. As they headed toward the kitchen, they passed by several pictures that were mounted on the wall. Curtis stopped to take a hard look at one of the pictures that caught his attention.

"My gosh! This man in the picture looks exactly like me."

Mable stopped, turned around, and headed back toward where Curtis was standing, looking at the picture. Her grocery bags still in his hands.

"Ah, yes," she said, taking the picture down from the wall.

"This is my dearly departed husband, Bobby. He died only a few years ago from cancer," Mable said, closing her eyes and hugging the picture close to her chest as a tear started to run down her cheek. Curtis placed the grocery bags down on the floor beside him and lifted his hand toward Mable to wipe the lone tear from her face. She looked up at Curtis and then down at the picture.

"Oh, Curtis, sweetheart, I am so sorry," she said, starting to cry. Both of them coming to the same conclusion.

"I must have made your life a living hell," she said, dropping her gaze to the floor.

"No, ma'am, you haven't," Curtis said, placing his fingers under her chin and lifting her face to meet his gaze.

"Actually, I'm honored. But I really do not believe in reincarnations, neither do I believe in anything of that sort, but I do understand."

"I am so glad that you do," Mable said, looking up at him, "Bobby's death has been so extremely hard on me, and I guess I was unconsciously grasping at straws, hoping that he had come back to me. For the life of me, it didn't click until just now."

"Ms. Kirkwood," Curtis said in a mock scolding tone, "now that everything has been cleared up, I never want to see you look like this again." Curtis pointed a finger at her, moving it up and down.

"You are a very beautiful woman, and you don't need any of this junk that you have on."

Mable smiled up at him and then returned the picture to where it was mounted. Curtis bent down to retrieve the grocery bags from the floor.

"Now, where do we put these?" he said, smiling down at her.

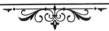

You're a Stinking Liar

Dana sat patiently in the patient's waiting area. She had already seen the doctor and was now waiting for the paratransit van to make its glorious appearance. She had about a good thirty minutes to kill before the van was due to arrive. So to kill the remaining minutes, she browsed over an edition of Better Homes and Gardens magazine.

Upon sifting through the well-worn pages, she found an interesting recipe for what was called Monkey Bread. Dana then asked the young lady sitting at the reception desk if it would be okay if she could tear the recipe out of the magazine. The young lady looked at her and asked, "What was the issue month?"

Dana flipped the magazine to its front cover and found the information that the young lady was requesting. The issue month as well as the year was found in the upper-left hand corner of the magazine.

"October 2013," Dana finally said, looking at the young woman in anticipation.

"Be my guest and rip away," the young lady said, smiling.

Dana smiled in return and politely said, "Thank you."

She then proceeded to carefully rip the recipe from the magazine. As she glanced over the recipe, she happily realized that she had all the ingredients on hand at home and decided she would give this oddly named concoction a try.

As Dana continued browsing through the magazine, trying to find more recipes she could obtain, she was totally unaware of the fact that more than thirty minutes had passed. The paratransit van had arrived, and the driver had slipped into the building and was roaming around looking for her.

"Ah, there you are, my sumptuous queen," the paratransit driver said upon spotting her, plastering a huge cheesy grin on his face.

"Oh, hey," Dana said, plastering on a quick and rather fake smile while trying to refrain from rolling her eyes.

"Please give me a few minutes," the paratransit driver said in his deep, rich Jamaican voice, "I have to go to the Mandinka Warrior's room, and I promise you honey boo, it won't take long at all."

"That will be fine, Kwesi. Please take as long as you need," Dana said, gathering up her things and sucking back up the overwhelming feeling of sadness because her prayer of Lord-I-don't-want-to-see-Kwesi-today went unanswered.

"Excuse me, ma'am," the young woman behind the reception desk said once the paratransit driver was out of earshot, "did you really just call that nice-looking man crazy to his face?"

"No," Dana said, laughing, "I said Kwesi. He told me a while ago that his name is spelled K-w-e-s-I, and it is pronounced Kway-zee."

"Oh, for a minute there, I thought you were about to start something."

"Ha," Dana blurted out, "no, not me. Although if I did, I think I could take him."

"Um, if you don't mind, will you allow me to do that instead," the young woman said with a mischievous look on her face.

"Be my guest," Dana said, "but please beware. I think that there is something fishy about him, and for the life of me, I can't quite figure it out yet."

"My precious angel, thank you so much for waiting for me," Kwesi said upon his return, rudely interrupting the conversation between the young women.

"Like I had any other choice but to wait," Dana mumbled under her breath. She then turned to face the young receptionist to wave goodbye and mouthed, "He is all yours if you want him, but buyer beware."

Dana stepped into the paratransit van, and Kwesi closely followed in behind her.

"Since you didn't allow me to carry your bags for you, please allow me to do the honor of buckling your seat belt," Kwesi said, following Dana deeper into the bus.

"Oh, no thank you. Believe me, I got it," Dana said, sitting down on the closest available seat. She quickly grabbed the belt and pulled it across her waist and locked it into position.

"Tsk, tsk, tsk," Kwesi said. "You adorable, strong African American women, and your I'm every woman pride," Kwesi said, bending down and unlocking Dana's seat belt. He adjusted the belt so that it would fit a little tighter across her waist. *That was totally and beyond unnecessary,* Dana wanted to tell him as she inhaled his overpowering cologne, the name of which had to have been Perry Smellus.

As she sat there watching the driver taking his sweet time buckling her back in, she noticed that he had unbuttoned the top two buttons of his uniform shirt, revealing what looked like a thick gold chain with splashes of booger-green coloring on it. He must have unbuttoned his shirt in the Mandinka Warrior's room, whatever the Mandinka Warrior's room was.

"There we go, to the keeper of my heart," Kwesi said, slowly straightening back up, his face within inches of Dana's, "it would hurt me something awful if I made a hard turn, and you went flying out of your seat."

Dana looked up at him and forced a smile onto her face.

"Thank you for being so considerate and kind to me, Kwesi, but I'm a pro at this paratransit thing. I've been riding now for a few years, and I know what driver's drive like they are bats out of *H-E Double Hockey Sticks.* I know which ones I should immediately start calling on the name of Jesus Christ the second I lay eyes on them. I also know which ones I should grab onto something and hold on for dear life until I reach my destination. And you, sweetie, I don't have to worry about none of that, although I do say a quick prayer for traveling mercies. I honestly think that you are one of the safest drivers out here."

"Do you really mean that?"

"Yes, I do," Dana said, really meaning it.

Kwesi looked at her. His gaze then dropped to the floor. He began moving his foot as if he was pushing around a small piece of trash, but there was nothing there. He locked eyes with Dana one final time before turning around to head toward the driver's seat.

As Dana settled into her seat and as she watched as Kwesi pulled the paratransit van into traffic, she immediately became happy. She remembered that she had a bag of Frito Lay Chili Cheese Corn chips and a bottle of orange soda in her purse. She would not go hungry on this time-consuming trip.

History had proven time and time again that whenever she was cursed to have Kwesi pick her up, he almost never took her straight home. On more than one occasion, her average ride time was at least three hours long even before he made any attempt to take her home. And as always, during those trips, he never stopped trying to hook up with her. He asked her out constantly, always complimented her and always called her those silly little froufrou names. Sometimes it bugged her to no end, and she wanted to call into the office to have him written up. At other times, she got a huge kick out of how hard he was trying to impress her.

Honestly, Dana didn't think that Kwesi was a bad-looking guy. He was rather on the handsome side. He fit her height requirements, and he looked as if he visited a gym or two. Those dreadlocks of his definitely had to go, but other than that, he was okay. And for the first time since riding with Kwesi, she felt something pure and honest about him when she had complimented him on his driving skills. Whatever it was that Dana felt, seriously intrigued her, and she honestly wanted to find out more about this handsome Jamaican paratransit driver.

"Base to 082," the dispatcher said over the radio.

"This is 082," Kwesi said, speaking onto the radio's mouth piece.

"Mrs. Sanchez called and said that she is ready to be picked up now."

"Okay, base, I'm headed that way now. Hope you don't mind Dana-boo, but it looks like you are going to be on the van for a few more minutes." Dana stuffed a few more corn chips in her mouth before looking down at her watch. She was almost at the hour-and-a-half mark of riding on the van.

"Okay," she said, trying not to spew her combination lunch and dinner out of her mouth.

"I think you'll like Mrs. Sanchez. She is a nice lady and very personable, and I really like talking to her."

"That's cool," Dana said and continued under her breath, "I hope she can run some interference with you trying to date me." The other four passengers that Kwesi had picked up and dropped off were of no help to her cause at all, and she desperately needed the break from Kwesi's nonstop jaw boxing. Dana quietly thanked God for Mrs. Sanchez. But in spite of the madness of being on the paratransit van for almost two hours, for some odd reason, Dana was still holding on to that brief moment of purity and sweetness that Kwesi showed while still in her doctor's office parking lot.

She also noticed that when he was talking to the dispatcher, his heavy Jamaican accent sort of flickered away during the conversation which she thought was rather odd. Dana felt her senses heighten. She wasn't sure why, but she began to think that the Jamaican persona was nothing more than an act, and she had a funny feeling that things were about to blow up in a matter of minutes.

As Kwesi pulled up into the parking lot for Woodmans, he carefully navigated around rogue shopping carts and people who were not paying attention to what they were doing. He pulled up in front of the entrance way which was marked with a huge red letter *A*, and before he could come to a complete stop, a rather large woman came flying out of the door with a personal shopping cart in tow, yelling and screaming at the top of her lungs.

"It's about time you showed up!" The woman screamed as she drew closer to the paratransit van. Dana quickly put away her half-eaten bag of chips and her nearly empty bottle of soda into her purse. She then peered out of the window to see a woman throwing up her fists at the paratransit driver.

"Don't move," Kwesi directed his command to Dana without turning around to face her and then exited the vehicle. As Kwesi walked around the front of the paratransit van, Dana's eyes stayed fixed on him watching his every move. Her hand reached inside her purse's outside pocket to retrieve her cell phone. A few quick swipes across the face of the phone, and Dana's finger now hovered over the speed button for 911.

Dana saw Kwesi approach the woman, his hands raised in surrender, as he began to talk to the belligerent woman in an attempt to calm her down. Five minutes' worth of conversation later, Dana saw the woman turn, look directly at her, and then smile the creepiest smile Dana ever did see, which set Dana completely on edge. So much so that Dana moved to the rear of the paratransit van and took a seat closest to the rear emergency exit. Dana didn't know what was about to happen, but she wanted to be prepared in any case.

Upon his return, Kwesi hadn't noticed that Dana had moved to the rear of the van and out of harm's way. He appeared to be in his own little now-messed-up world.

"This is 082 to base."

"082, go."

"Base, I have Ms. Washington standing outside of my van wanting to get on. She said that she had been waiting here for over two hours for a van to pick her up."

"Oops," was the dispatcher's reply.

"What do you mean by oops?" Kwesi snapped back.

"Well, the driver of 102 was scheduled to pick her up, but um, Ms. Washington doesn't like that particular driver, and that driver despises Ms. Washington to no end. And in order to avoid conflict, we figured you could grab her and take her home especially since you were headed that way to pick up Mrs. Sanchez. Besides, we know she really likes you," the dispatcher said, laughing, along with several others that could be heard laughing in the background.

Gathering himself together, Kwesi took in an extremely deep breath before speaking, "Base, please transfer her information over to my tablet so I can take her home." A few seconds later, a confirmation beep could be heard on Kwesi's work tablet, and then Kwesi slowly opened the doors to the van. Dana sat back and took in all the action as her heart went out to Kwesi who, by the way, was completely talking without his Jamaican accent. However, in spite of the missing flavor to his voice, she really wanted to go to the front of the van and grab him and tell him that it would all be okay, but as she saw the huge black woman enter the door of the van. Dana froze in her seat.

"Hello, Ms. Pretty Thang," Ms. Washington said to Dana as she plopped into the seat closest to Kwesi.

"Girlfriend, why did you move?"

"If you really must know," Dana said in response, "I moved because I saw you acting like a mad dog out there. And God knows that I didn't want to get bitten and run the risk of needing to get shots for rabies."

"Oh, is that so!"

"Yes, it is," Dana said, snapping back and gaining strength from God only knew from where. Ms. Washington stood back to her feet and turned to face Dana. As she stood there, she eyed Dana from head to toe menacingly.

"I'm not threatened by you, Ms. Thang."

"My name is Dana," Dana said in a matter-of-fact tone, "and I've given you no reason to be threatened by me."

"That's right because you recognize who I am."

"Honestly, I couldn't care less about who you are, Ms. Washington. I have better things to occupy my time."

"Lisa!" Kwesi shouted out, "leave Dana alone and take your seat. I am picking up one more individual from this place, and as soon as she is buckled in, I am taking you straight home."

"Okay, my sweet baby boo," Ms. Washington said, taking her seat and buckling herself in.

"Lisa, we have been over this time and time again. There is nothing between us and nor will there ever be."

"Come on now, Keith."

"Keith!" Dana yelled out in confusion.

"Ha, has my boo been lying again and saying that he is from Jamaica and his name is Kwesi?" Lisa said, laughing.

"Shame on you, Keith!"

"Keith, my dear," Mrs. Sanchez said stepping onto the Paratransit van. She handed her fare, which was three dollars, over to the driver.

"I know that this is asking a lot, but would you mind terribly if I was the first one you dropped off?"

"I'll see what I can do," Keith said rather somberly.

"I hope you two ladies don't mind if Keith bends the rules a little," Mrs. Sanchez said as she sat down in the seat once occupied by Dana. Lisa immediately began laughing as she turned to face Dana.

"It looks like you were the only one that didn't know that his name was Keith!" Lisa said, rocking back and forth in her seat. She was laughing so hard that it became difficult for her to catch her breath. As Dana sat there, watching whatever *his* name was help Mrs. Sanchez into her seat. A mixture of conflicting emotions overcame her.

She didn't know whether to scream or to take aim and throw her purse. She also didn't know whether or not to take the initiative and permanently stop Ms. Lisa Washington from laughing. Dana immediately came to herself and quickly repented for her thoughts of murder. *Lord, I'm sorry,* She thought to herself. *You said in your word, you can get angry but sin not.*

As Dana sat there in her seat, she turned her head to glance out of the window. As she peered at the shoppers coming in and out of Woodmans, she made up in her mind that she didn't want to know why Kwesi or Keith lied. All she wanted to do was go home and fix her Monkey Bread.

She had felt some time ago that there was something fishy about this dude. Now, she knew for sure that this guy was a no good stinking liar, and she would have no more to do with him. As Keith finished up buckling in Mrs. Sanchez, he took one final glance at Dana as a lone tear fell from one of his eyes. He then turned around to head to the driver's seat, but before he made it there, he heard someone scream

"*Callete!*" An immediate hush fell over the van as Keith quickly turn around to face his passengers. He saw Mrs. Sanchez pointing a weary finger at Lisa, and she screamed once again, "*Callete!* You evil, no good woman. Keith told me about you, how evil and malicious you were to him."

For confirmation, Mrs. Sanchez turned to look at Keith and saw him nod his head.

"You tried to ruin this young man's life with your lies, and with your stalking him," Mrs. Sanchez continued, her eyes once again fixed on Lisa.

"He moved from Chicago to Rockford to get away from you, and you followed him here. What in the world made you think that he wanted you. For heaven's sake, you are forty years older than he is, old enough to be his mother. Yet and still, you kept insisting on trying to entice and seduce him. He also told me about you," Mrs. Sanchez said, turning to face Dana.

"For goodness' sake, this boy lights up every time he talks about you. The reason why he lied sweetie was to protect you."

"To protect—" Dana started to say, but Mrs. Sanchez lifted a hand to gently silence her.

"This thing over here," she said pointing a finger at Lisa, "chased away the last young lady he liked. She even went as far as to threaten her very life, which I know for a fact because I had the opportunity to talk with her before she moved to Texas. She wasn't any good for him anyway," she said, throwing a quick glance at Keith.

"But you, *hija mia*, this boy is in love with you. He gave you a false name so that he would feel safe to date you. And if this thing over here ever approached you, you would be safe in saying that your boyfriend was from Jamaica and his name was Kwesi. It wasn't until this woman found out where he worked and paid someone to injure her so that she could qualify to ride paratransit when she found out his pseudo identity."

As Mrs. Sanchez continued to explain the details to Dana, no one noticed that Lisa had unbuckled her seat belt. In a matter of seconds, she hefted herself across the aisle and began to choke Mrs. Sanchez. Keith ran and grabbed Lisa by her blouse and yanked her back, slamming her into the rear of the driver's seat. Dana quickly unbuckled her seat belt and ran up to check on Mrs. Sanchez.

"I'm okay, *hija mia*," Mrs. Sanchez said in a raspy voice. As Keith turned to focus his attention on Mrs. Sanchez, Lisa grabbed hold of one of the seat belt extensions that was hanging on the wall of the paratransit van. As she turned, she extended her arm, and the buckle of the belt slammed hard into Keith's back. He yelled out in pain as he grabbed at his back and tumbled to the floor. Without thinking, Dana maneuvered carefully over Keith and then charged at Lisa. She slammed her body hard into Lisa's, causing the van to rock from side to side; the force of it caused one of the van's windows to shatter into pieces.

Instinctively, Dana grabbed at one of the broken shards still clinging on to its frame and quickly moved it near Lisa's carotid artery.

"I dare you!" Dana said through clenched teeth.

Keith pushed the chair under Dana as she slowly eased down. After he made sure she was comfortable, he took a couple of steps and sat down in the chair directly across from her.

"Have you eaten here before?" Keith said nervously.

"Actually, no, I haven't. But when we walked into the door, the aroma of the cooking food caused my mouth to water." They exchanged a fleeting glance at each other as the waitress approached their table.

"Welcome to Famous Daves. I'm Famous Monica, may I start you off with some drinks?"

"Yes," Keith said, "I'll have a raspberry iced tea."

"And how about you, young lady?" the waitress said, turning to Dana, "I'll have a Mountain Dew if you have it."

"Why, yes, we do," the waitress said, "I'll be back with your drinks in just a sec."

"You know," Dana said, partially glancing over the menu, "Mrs. Sanchez should be here with us."

"She is, in a way," Keith said rather coyly.

"What do you mean?"

Keith smiled as he whipped out the gift card and said, "She's paying for our first date."

"That sweet old lady," Dana said, shaking her head from side to side.

"Dana," Keith now said, his voice serious, "why wouldn't you—" But before he could finish his sentence, Dana interrupted him.

"Because my Spidey senses were tingling."

Keith looked at her, confused.

"The last guy that I dated lied so much that in a way, he trained me how to pick up on subtle clues to alert me to when someone was lying. And um, you're not a good liar," Dana said, smiling.

"I am so sorry—"

"Don't even worry about it," Dana said, cutting him off, "Lisa Washington is locked up and has been charged with assault with a deadly weapon and attempted murder. Mrs. Sanchez is paying for dinner. You will be released to go back to work in a couple of weeks. And I am on a date with a very handsome man named Keith who I am going to enjoy getting to know."

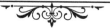

Look Out Fixed Route

Usually when I catch wind that a particular driver wants to transfer over to the RMTD fixed-route side, I'm not a happy camper. I sometimes show my discontentment and try to convince the driver that he and/or she should stay with paratransit. I usually scream out, "Why in the world would you do such a horrible thing!"

But honestly, I already know the reason why they want to transfer over. It's all about the Benjamins. In their world, there are tall mountains covered with greenbacks in all sorts of denominations, fountains crafted by heavenly angels, that instead of water springing out of them, silver and bronze coins pop up out of their silver-plated spouts.

When it rains, the drivers use their company-paid umbrellas crafted out of American Express gold cards to protect them from the terminal to their buses. Well, I am exaggerating quite a bit, but money is indeed a reason why I lose some awesome paratransit drivers. Another reason why I believe that they transfer over to the dark side is that they can move up the ranks a little quicker. With both sides, you start out part-time, but I think you make it to a full-time position quicker than you would on the paratransit side.

Although it amazes me to this day, more money on the fixed-route side, but more work on the paratransit side. Go figure! Honestly, I don't fault the drivers for wanting to get ahead and find more solid ground to stand on. However, I personally feel that I have lost some really good drivers. Although on occasion, I do get to see them from time to time.

On this particular day, I met the worse paratransit driver in my young life. I never thought I would ever say and/or wish for someone to transfer over to the fixed-route side, but that all came to a shattering halt when I met, well, I'll just call him Mr. DooWacky.

I am not going to go into details as to what Mr. DooWacky looks like because that's not important. Just know that I am blessed as well as thankful that he has decided to go over to the fixed-route side. I am quite sure that other passengers maybe just as happy as I am about his decision.

On one of my excursions, I did overhear one passenger refer to Mr. DooWacky as being a fool and that he would probably get killed on the fixed-route side. That remains to be seen; nothing in the news yet. But honestly, I would really hate for any driver to get hurt and especially killed. That just simply wouldn't be cool. And no, I wouldn't want anything like that to happen to Mr. DooWacky except for him maybe getting suspended from driving for a couple of weeks or so.

Anyway, I had scheduled a double ride for the day that I was unfortunate enough to run into Mr. DooWacky. Surprisingly enough, it was my first time meeting him, and I thank God that it would also be my last time riding on a paratransit van with him. He pulled up in front of destination number one thirteen minutes ahead of schedule. Now normally, I am flexible. I usually try to stop what I am doing and try to accommodate the paratransit drivers. I do realize and understand that they are sometimes running tight schedules. They are sometimes expected to get from one side of town to the next in two minutes flat with time to spare.

Granted, I have been on those vans where I've had to hold on for dear life where the driver did indeed make it across town in two minutes. On this day, however, which was marred by Mr. DooWacky, I did call an early end to what I was doing and headed out to get on the van.

Strike number one. When I arrived at the door, he mentioned that he was just about to call into the office on me. I guess I was taking too long to come out to the van, and he wanted them to rush me along. I had thirteen minutes left before my scheduled pick up time, and if I just simply wanted to sit on my hands and rock from side to side, I was well within my rights to do so. My pickup time was 1:30, not 1:17. I know it was only thirteen minutes, but Mr. DooWacky made me mad.

Strike number two. Anyone that is not a smoker, me being included in that bunch, can easily pick up on faint traces of cigarette smoke or any other kind of smoke for that matter. I don't know why, but there seems to be an extra sensitivity that the nose has.

Ha, there was no need for the extra senses to kick in on this day. Mr. DooWacky's van was completely and totally lit up. I'm saying to myself, *Oh my heaven, this van stinks*. There weren't enough open windows to dissipate the stench from his smoking. Now, I had no idea whether or not he stepped off the van to light up and quickly got back on the bus. Nor did I know if he simply opened the driver side window to catch a few quick puffs before I showed up, but in either case, it was just wrong. In all my time riding with paratransit, I have never been on a van that stank like that. Not even from being on the van with someone that was picked up from the "Y" after a strenuous workout. I honestly couldn't believe how that van smelled, especially since I had never been on a van that reeked of cigarette smoke before. Mr. DooWacky was quickly headed down hill in my book.

Strike number three, which is not the final strike, but it was indeed one of the worse. Mr. DooWacky had enough nerve to start talking about some of the other paratransit drivers. As far as I was concerned that was and shall forever be a big no-no. On this day, I was looking at him, thinking to myself, *I have been riding longer than you have been driving so how dare you fix your mouth to talk about another driver, especially since you just arrived on the paratransit scene.*

One particular driver that came into the discussion, and I tried my best to suggest to Mr. DooWacky that maybe they were going through something personal and that they maybe just didn't quite know how to deal with what they were going through. And that maybe he was coming to work and inadvertently taking out his frustration out on his fellow coworkers. Mr. DooWacky had no sympathy whatsoever.

Granted, I realize that if a person is having personal problems, they should keep it in check and not spew it out like pea soup, like that woman did in the movie *The Exorcist*. But Mr. DooWacky showed that he personally did not have a heart. He told me that particular driver hated him and he hated him in return. However, he didn't provide any proof whatsoever that the other driver hated him.

There were two other drivers that came into the discussion, and I guess Mr. DooWacky was trying to feel me out on them. He actually asked me how did I feel about them. The two drivers that he brought up, I actually like and would defend them if need be. As a matter of fact, I even like the one he said that he hated. But nevertheless, I spoke positively concerning the other two drivers that he had placed on his chopping block. I guess since I talked positively concerning them, it forced him to do the same. I knew what game he was trying to play, and it stank just like the van did. You don't mess with my paratransit drivers, especially those that I carry in my heart.

Strike number four. GPS can be your friend, but it also can be your enemy. But if you need GPS to get to where you need to go, by all means, allow the thing to talk to you. I guess pride was an issue that Mr. DooWacky suffered from on this day. If he would have allowed the GPS system to talk to him and not use it on the down low, everything would have been cool.

Now what I am about to say is very sad. When Mr. DooWacky picked me up, he informed me that he had another passenger that he had to pick up and drop off before he took me to my second destination. I was cool with it, no biggie. Things like this happens when you ride paratransit. Anyway, the individual that he had to pick up wasn't too far from where I boarded the van, and where they needed to go was maybe a mile or so from where they were picked up.

Nevertheless, Mr. DooWacky couldn't find it even with using GPS. Now, if Mr. DooWacky had the GPS operating to where he could have listened to the nice voice, it clearly would have stated that his destination was on the right. After hearing the other passenger speak, even I knew where they needed to go. I even chimed in and told him exactly where the building was. So Mr. DooWacky looped around and did something that was totally unsafe as well as illegal

Instead of making a complete pass around to where he would be able to drop the passenger off properly, he made a turn which placed him on an angle in front of the curb that was to the left of the destination. This act of laziness left the rear end of the paratransit van sticking out into the street. Now this wasn't your normal run-of-the-mill residential street. It was a major, highly congested street—one of the busiest streets in Rockford. I thank God that nothing big and bad came down that street that could have clipped the back end clean, taking along with it the back wheels and me for that matter.

You may be wondering why I didn't call in to report Mr. DooWacky. Well, let me tell you. First of all, this guy would have considered it a badge of honor. He probably would have gone around boasting and bragging that he got written up for simply doing his job. I say poo-poo to that idea. Second, he stated, while I was on the van, that he was written up before; it wasn't his first time, and it probably wouldn't be his last. Although how we got on that topic of discussion, I haven't the foggiest idea. Besides, who goes around bragging about something like that anyway? Finally, I am not a rat. I turn the problems that I have with the drivers, if any, over to a higher power.

Anyway, God has moved him to the fixed-route side, and I really don't have to deal with, look at, and/or even smell him anymore. Let fixed-route deal with him, and I'm quite sure that they will. Besides, this dude was so cocky that he will definitely make his presence known. So farewell Mr. DooWacky. I am so glad that you are no longer a paratransit driver.

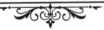

Paratransit Newbies

First and foremost, please allow me to apologize to you because the following set of stories is being written in anger and frustration. Now before you close the book and slam it on your coffee table, or even better still, the dashboard of the paratransit van, please allow me to explain myself.

We all have those precious moments where we want to slap someone upside their head to possibly knock some sense into them. We may even want to gently choke them to get the stupid out of them. Please don't get me wrong. I do not, and I repeat, I do not want to kill them. The only thing that I really want to do is maybe just do a little damage and have their faces marked for a couple of weeks or so to let the world know that they were beyond wrong.

Believe me, I know that some of you are in agreement with me because some of the stories I've heard of what you want to do to an individual, whoa! So let's agree that I won't tell on you and you won't tell on me, okay? So far, I haven't hit anyone, but again, it is not like I don't want to. The odds are extremely great, however, that I won't even lift my pinky finger, but sometimes, I just want to handle my business.

The following stories are about three separate individuals. I doubt that you will be able to figure out who they are, so don't even try. I know that you are probably still racking your brain about who in the world wrote this book of short stories about the exciting world of paratransit. Just let it go, okay? Because I promise you will never figure it out. Just know that I am Ms. Sara Rockford, and that is all you are getting out of me, well besides these stories.

But anyhow, these three individuals I do care about, some more than others. So in a way, I will try my best to be somewhat gentle in describing what happened that made me want to punch them. But in all honesty, I hope that you are able to get a laugh out of what is being written. This will definitely let you know that passengers can be just as irritating and annoying as some of the drivers as well as those people who work in the office. What makes these stories and/ or individuals unique? They are all newbies to the wonderful and exciting world of paratransit. So please, sit back and enjoy!

I will start off with the worse of the three individuals. This person is really sweet. She can be a little obnoxious at times. She can also be a little chatty Kathy, so I would recommend you purchasing some good quality earplugs. But after a while, she can grow on you, but you have to be careful that she doesn't turn out to be one of those vines that cover some of the buildings here in Rockford. Actually, I think that those things are rather hideous, but I digress. So you may be asking, "What makes me want to slap this individual?" Well, let me tell you.

Now I do not believe that this person has been riding paratransit for no more than a year. Probably not even that long, so all their experiences riding on the vans are so fresh and exciting to them, especially the drivers. But that is a different story. One in which you will read about much later. I promise you.

I have been riding paratransit for a wee bit longer than they have. So I know some of the ins and outs, some of the driver's names, and yes, some of their work schedules; which, by the way, comes in awful handy when you want to avoid a specific driver. I've done it, and in a way, I am still doing it. But please forgive me, I am slipping into yet another story. They are just flowing out of me like liquid gold.

Anyway, I kind of advised them to get to know the drivers because it is good to know who is picking you up for several reasons. For one, you will know how to pray. Another reason why is that you will know, by the driver, that you need to hurry up and sit down. You will then need to buckle up and get that seat belt as tight as you can get it across your waist and grab on to anything you can that is within reach and don't let go until it is your turn to get off the van. Sometimes, posted speed limits mean nothing to these drivers. I'm a witness. Another reason is that you can develop some really good friendships as I have.

Did they take my advice? You may be asking? Well, yes, they did. However, they became fixated on one particular driver. For the sake of this story, I'll just call him Matthew. Now, I will admit that Matthew is beyond delicious-looking. He is a little on the vertically challenged side, but his looks as well as his personality more than make up for his height deficiency.

Personally, I like Matthew, but I'm not envisioning him walking down the aisle with me and having two and a half kids with him. Now moving right along to the irritating part, believe it or not, I somehow ended up on Para-Matthew Watch. What do I mean by Para-Matthew Watch? Well let me explain it to you since you asked.

As previously stated, I ride paratransit more than they do, and sometimes in conversations, I let them know that I'm going out. So when they think that I have made it back home, I get a text asking who my drivers were. I honestly thought the whole point in utilizing the paratransit service is getting from point A to point B and them back to point A. Am I right? I know you can't answer me directly, but what you can do is close your eyes for about two seconds and subliminally send me a message telling me that I am indeed right.

Now this has happened more than I care to admit. Since they don't ride as often as I do, they are hoping that I will run into Matthew. Then if I do, I can give them the full report. What did he smell like? Were there any other passengers on the van with you? Did he take you straight home? What did you talk about? Did you mention me? My goodness! Before writing this story, the last time that I went out on paratransit and they knew about it, I had two female drivers. When they sent me a text asking who my drivers were, I told them the name of one of the girls and that I didn't know the name of the other young lady. But I wanted to add, "Ha, how do you like those, garbanzo beans? It wasn't Matthew."

Please forgive me for the use of profanity just now. Garbanzo beans is a strong curse word, and I shouldn't have used it. So please, for my sake, just throw your hands up into the air and say, "Lord, bless her."

It is a shame that I am being pestered about who my drivers are whenever I go out. It is also a shame that I have gotten to the point where I even don't want to run into Matthew. I am literally two steps away from asking God to make this a reality. Again, Matthew is super cool and super sexy, but I don't want to get hit with a barrage of questions if I run into him by this sweet individual. When you think about it, even though I may ride paratransit more, we still have about the same chance of running into Matthew.

Actually, riding paratransit is like the deadly game Russian roulette because you have no idea of what driver is coming to pick you up. Right now, you may be asking, why tell them that I'm riding paratransit anyway? Gosh, darn, good question! But when the text messages come through, asking me, "Did you go anywhere today?" What am I supposed to say? You try telling someone in a nice way that what they are asking is none of their business, and it really doesn't matter.

Although the very last time they sent me a text message, I wanted to find them and smash my phone on their face. I took my sweet time telling them who my drivers were for a particular day, and would you believe, they sent me a text back saying, "Drivers please." And to top it off, there was an exclamation mark at the end of the word *please*. A part of me was screaming, *Girl, you need a life.* The other part was screaming, *Really?*

Nevertheless, let's see how far you get without sounding rude and making a sweet person run into a corner and start balling their eyes out. So I guess the irritation will continue until either they marry Matthew or they stop liking him altogether, which for right now is highly unlikely.

Now this next person, I simply just want to punch in the throat and possibly knock some humbleness into. Normally, I am not a violent person, but right now, I am at the edge. The shocker about this person is that he/she doesn't even ride paratransit. Honestly, I don't think that he/she has ever been on a paratransit van. What could be irritating about he/she you may be asking? Wow, you are asking some really good questions. And let me answer you.

Have you ever been around a person who wanted to appear more knowledgeable than what they really are? I believe we have all had those moments where we have felt a little bit inadequate, maybe even out of place. But I have learned that if you don't' know something, admit to it and don't seek out ways to make yourself appear to be bigger and smarter than what you really are and make it appear that you know it all, especially if the information you are seeking is of no real use to you. *And* the only reason why you are asking for the information is again to make yourself seem more knowledgeable to the person who you are in turn passing the information on to.

I know that I have said a lot, and it may be a little confusing, so allow me to break it down to you. This person, I'll just call her Robin was pumping me for information concerning paratransit. They were not asking for the information for themselves. They were asking for a friend of theirs whose brother is starting to ride.

Now do you see just how many unnecessary people are involved in this little scenario. Common sense, why can't the one who will be riding paratransit call into the office to get the information that he needs? You would think that this would be the case, but no, Robin is asking me all kinds of questions only to appear in front of her friend to be well versed in the knowledge of paratransit. Really! Is it that serious!

Besides, good old-fashioned common sense would let you know that something could have easily been omitted as well as added in the passing along of information from one person to the next. For example, I can tell person A that a particular guy is cute. Person A may tell person B that not only do I think this guy is cute but I also like him. Person B may tell person C that I am six months pregnant with this guy's baby. By the time we get down to person Z, I'm a suspect in this guy's murder because I became jealous of him dating my best friend, and all I initially said was that he was cute. I know that this may be a bit extreme, but do you get my point? You are a smart person, so I know you understand.

I hope that you agree with me that Robin should mind her own business and simply tell her friend's brother to call the paratransit office for himself. I also hope that you agree with me that Robin should stop trying to pump herself up and be content in the skin that she is in. Yes, knowledge is power, and yes, people perish for a lack of knowledge. But she doesn't even ride paratransit, nor do I think she ever will. And I really do not know of any one person that knows or should know everything. If you know of anyone that does and should, again with the subliminal thing, please let me know.

Finally, I'm down to the last one in this trio of paratransit newbies. This person you may have some sympathy for after reading this short story and, if you do good, for you. You are all right in my book, literally, ha! However, what can I say to describe this situation? Well, I will try to be as gentle in telling this story as I possibly can. Because when you really think about it, they are just innocent. They didn't know. But still, smack, smack across the face. In reality, they should have known better.

Here is something to think about. If a storm rolls through Rockford, what could possibly happen? Please don't say duh because you know as well as I know that some of everything and anything could happen if and when a storm hits anywhere, any place at any time. It can be potentially dangerous and life-threatening. People's lives can be changed drastically. You never really can tell what can or what will happen. Pretty much all you can do is pray and hope for the best if and when a storm does hit. I have been blessed, however. During my time living here in Rockford, I haven't had the experience of being in a bad storm. Granted, I have heard sirens going off from time to time, but nothing really major except for hard rain which leads me into the next story.

A good rainstorm, in any area, can knock a few things out of whack. But this particular rainstorm, which happened a few days ago, knocked out the phone lines to the Rockford Mass Transit District building. This wasn't anything new to me. I have dealt with this type of thing before in the past, and I'm quite sure I will have to deal with it again in the future. It is a part of the ordeal of having to utilize public transportation. No biggie, or so it would seem, at least to me anyway.

Well anyhow, I received a call from a person who was trying to call into paratransit to schedule a ride for someone. They called me asking me why they were not able to get through. Now, this person knows that I have been riding for a while and probably figured that I am the resident paratransit expert. No, not by a long shot, and nor do I want to be either. But again, they called me asking me why couldn't they get through. Really? I guess this was the first initial thought that came to my mind. But after I gathered myself together and instead of being condescending, I began to explain to them the reason why I thought that they couldn't get through. I figured that it was because of the heavy rain. And boy, did it really come down that day. I also told them that I was also trying to get through for myself. I reassured them that something like this happens all the time and to keep trying until they were able to get through.

Yes, I was nice to them as I should have been. And in their defense, they were originally from Chicago. Now we all know that Rockford can fit inside Chicago a few times over. And I am quite sure that in the greater Chicago land area that there are backup generators to the backup generators. And it would take a whole lot of rain to knock anything out in that humongous city. But still! I'll think I will just leave it at that and publicly proclaim and declare that I am not the resident paratransit expert. I guess I will also be there again for them if they have any more paratransit questions.

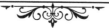

Compassion

Believe it or not, not all the passengers who utilize the paratransit services are born with their respective disabilities. There are a numbered few of us whose lives were sucker punched. Either through no fault of our own and maybe even through fault of our own, we were thrusted into a world we never wanted to be in. Nor did we ever imagine that our lives would take such a drastic turn.

Being short on cash or being in a horrible relationship with someone is part of life's norm, but having to adjust to a different lifestyle after being declared disabled, excuse my French, really bites. For those of us who are the recently disabled, our stories are unique. The people who I have met who have joined the disabled club, their stories would surprise and shock quite a few of you. I will let you in on a few of those stories, but you can forget about me telling you mine because it may disclose who I am.

Diabetes is a common cause of a number of things, and in some cases, the cause of a person's disability. There are also other health issues that would affect a person's life as well as their livelihood, such as high blood pressure, cancer, tumor, and the like.

One young man, who I thought was simply adorable, said that a dog scratched him in one of his eyes which caused him to lose his vision. Another individual who I was fortunate to meet in a class that I was blessed to take, was hit by a car; I believe during his senior year of high school. Now he is disfigured and walks with a cane. Yet another individual was attacked and beaten with a crowbar and spent a week in the hospital in a coma.

Just imagine being around him when the doctors told him his bad news. Granted, I'm quite sure that he was thankful because he was still numbered among the living, but still. As far as my own personal disability, again, I'm not going to tell you. I guess that you thought I was going to slip up at this emotional moment, but no. Just keep reading. You will see me pour out my heart as well as maintain my silence as to who I really am.

I haven't had a clue as to what these newly disabled people desire or thinking about. Each individual has their own personal story, their own personal journey, so I can only speak for myself. As far as I am concerned, I want the life I had before I became disabled. I wasn't rich or anything like that, but I was doing okay. I was able to get out and hang with friends and family, go where I wanted to go, and do what I wanted to do.

Granted, I still have somewhat of an active life, and I truly thank God for it, but it hurts to look at pictures of family and friends enjoying their lives to the fullest on social media outlets, and all I can do is look at the pictures and silently wish I was there with them having fun. I have nieces and nephews that I have never met. There have been weddings, even in my own family, that I would have loved to have attended the ceremony. I get invited to a lot of activities and events that I simply can't go to because of my disability and my inability to get out and travel like a normal person would. But again, I am thankful that I can at least see the pictures on social media. I am also thankful that every now and then, a friend or family member would send me a text message with a picture attached.

Now, you are probably wondering what in the world all of what was previously mentioned has to do with paratransit. I'm glad that your curiosity was peeked. If I had my life back, there would be no need for me to use paratransit, and I would have never met you, people. Now I know that sounds a little harsh, and honestly, I'm not trying to be that way. However, I have heard it said before: "What you never knew, you would never miss."

Due to my disability, I have formed some awesome friendships with some of the paratransit drivers. I even like a few people in the office. But if time could be turned back for me, and I'm quite sure a few other people who ride, we would be nice, productive people. Not to mention, we wouldn't have gotten on your nerves, and neither you on ours. Our paths would have never crossed. I could be completely wrong on the following point, but I'm almost positive that there are a few of you out there who wish you had never met me.

Again, what does this have to do with riding paratransit? Well, it is based on how we are sometimes treated by you guys and how we sometimes treat you. I know of this one young man, who shall remain nameless, wanted me to come to his apartment and read all the scriptures in the Bible where Jesus healed blinded eyes. I also think that he wanted to hook up with me, but I digress. But this young man falls into the category of the newly disabled. I have run into him at social events, and I have also been on the same paratransit van at times with him.

Unlike me, who cries and repents and asks God for restoration, he lashes out at people. And I am positive that he has verbally mowed down a few of you guys. He is quick to cop an attitude and tell you where to go and the shortest possible route of you getting there. I have also seen him on the paratransit van with his head bowed, deep in his own world. During those times, I wanted to grab him and hold him and tell him, "Baby, it will be okay."

So I have made it my business that whether or not I run into him at a social event or even on a paratransit van, I will give him a kiss on his cheek. Sometimes, the smallest gesture of kindness can cause a person to soar and stop an angry person from exploding. And sometimes, you paratransit people makes being disabled more difficult than what it should be. I can understand why sometimes, that young man that was previously mentioned lashes out at you guys even though he really shouldn't.

You are probably wondering how in the world I arrived at this conclusion. Well, let me tell you. The individuals who were born with their disabilities have an edge. They know how to roll with the punches. They can even throw some back. They can also laugh at themselves. But in my case, and I'm quite sure for others as well, all we can think about is I want my life back, and I wish that I didn't have to ride that white van because some of you drivers, as well as the office people, are not so nice to us.

Please allow me to give you a few examples of what I am talking about. I hope that with these examples you will have a better understanding of some of the challenges that we face on a day-to-day basis. Possibly, it may even help you to stop judging us and be a little bit more considerate as well as compassionate. Because, again, we were sucker punched into this lifestyle.

I had a conversation with one of the drivers, and they mentioned how they hated that the passengers called into the office asking where they were when they were running behind schedule. Because it is not like calling in would and or could force the drivers to get to a particular location any quicker than when they will actually arrive. I guess he feels that he is being pestered.

In a way because of what he said, I try my best not to call in asking where the paratransit van is when they are running behind schedule. But there were times where my hand was forced, and I had to call the office, and I am glad that I did.

You can learn a lot when you call. One particular time, I was waiting for the paratransit van to show up. I call myself patiently waiting, but time kept ticking by. When I eventually did call the office, the individual who I spoke to lied and said that I called the office and cancelled my ride. Now why would I be walking back and forth to the window looking for a van that I knew wasn't going to show up? And why would I call the office asking where is the paratransit van if I actually canceled my ride for the day? That doesn't even make good, stupid sense!

Another instance where my hand was forced to call the office was when I was waiting on paratransit to pick me up from a class I was attending in a building that was located just outside downtown Rockford. I was standing there waiting. It was cold. Snow and ice was on the ground, and everyone else in the class, including the teacher, had left for the evening. I called in and found out that I was on no one's paperwork for a return trip home.

Thank God I called because whoever it was dispatched a van to take me home. After talking to the driver, I found out that he was the last driver out for the night, and he was headed to the terminal. If I hadn't called, I would have been stranded.

Granted, this wasn't the only incident where if I hadn't called in to find out where the van was, I would have been stranded. I was at the Y, being trained on how to use the computer that kept track of a person's workout schedule. I later learned that the driver pulled up way before my scheduled pickup time and saw that I was engaged with an activity. They themselves called the office to say that I wasn't ready and asked for permission to pull off and leave me.

No one called me to let me know that the paratransit van had showed up. By default, I was thrown into standby mode which I didn't know that I was in. I believe God dispatched an angel just for me that walked up to me and said, "You have been waiting here a long time. You should call and check on your ride."

When I finally did call that is when I found out everything. I have several other stories I could tell you that if I hadn't called the office, I would have been screwed. To that paratransit driver who hates passengers calling in the office, checking on where they are at, what do you want me to do?

Granted, I realize that you do not have any superpowers and that you are doing the best that you can do. But when you say stuff like that, it only makes me wish all the more that I didn't need you guys and that I wasn't disabled. To call or not to call, that was the question.

I apologize for this particular story not being as humorous as the rest of the ones in this book. But you have to realize that your words as well as your actions can cause more damage to an already damaged person. This is not only directed at the drivers but to those of you who work in the office. We, I, the multitude really don't want to be the way that we are. And sometimes, you make life a little bit more difficult than what it should be. Sometimes, I know that it is done out of ignorance. But sometimes, I know that it is done on purpose.

If you were in my newly acquired disabled shoes, you would have a little bit more compassion. I'm quite sure that a number of you are saying, "Well, since you have such a problem with us, stop riding." Well, if I had a rich relative to pass away and leave me all their money, I would throw up the deuces sign in a heartbeat, and I would be free from the bonds of paratransit, and I promise you that I would not look back. So for this brief moment, if you have your virtual boxing gloves on, I have mine on as well.

In all fairness, I know that you guys are not the reason why I am disabled. You also had no clue as to who I was before I became disabled. Simply stated, you are just one of the reasons why I hate being disabled. You are a constant, extra reminder of my current state of being. I know that it may seem like that I am bashing you guys, but I'm really not. I am simply just stating hard, true facts. I am also trying to liberate you. Even the Bible states that the truth shall make you free.

Being free is a lovely state to be in. I also must point out that you all are in my prayers. And an elite few of you, if you need it, will get first dibs on a kidney, a lung, a few drops of blood, and even a bone marrow. I also want you all to look at things from a different perspective and just imagine if things were different if you were in my shoes.

For those of you who actually thought in your heads and maybe even vocalized it: "Just stop riding paratransit!" Well, just so you know, paratransit is not my only mode of transportation around Rockford. But even in someone else's car, you are still bound by rules and regulations. And sometimes, the ride itself is actually worse than riding paratransit. And before you can say nothing can make this woman happy, allow me to give you examples of what I am talking about.

Have you ever been in a car with someone who turned on their radio and started singing in a musical key that only they can sing in? For those of you who don't know, that musical key is called Z flat. For all of you musically inclined people, the highest note on any musical instrument you can play is in the key of G. You can't tell them to shut up because it is their car, and they are doing you a favor.

Or have you ever been in a car with someone and their "Aunt Gertrude" calls asking the person who is driving you around to do something for them? And because it is their Aunt Gertrude and they love Aunt Gertrude, you are rerouted, and by the time you get the ice cream that you have been craving home, it has turned into ice cream soup. I could go on, but I won't. I think that I have cried enough in writing this short story, and it is time to laugh again.

Please forgive me for not making you laugh and/or chuckle with this one particular short story, but I had to get the hurt and the pain off my chest. Yes, God has blessed, and he is still blessing. The Lord and savior definitely knows what he is doing, but I am still encased in this flesh, and somedays, I simply do not have the strength to simply just grin and bear it. Although, praise God, I'm getting better. But if I had the ability to turn back the hands of time, I would definitely be saying Para-What?

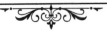

The Hated Driver

Although many of the Rockford citizens enjoyed the services that are offered by the paratransit division of the Rockford Mass Transit District (RMTD), Megan Sims was not numbered among that group. Granted, what person would not love to be greeted by a friendly, well-groomed, and good-smelling driver arriving in a clean, well-maintained city vehicle that offered door-to-door service.

One could easily find this a luxury, especially only having to pay a small meager amount of six dollars for a round-trip ride. The convenience of being shuttled anywhere your heart desired, within the Rockford city limits of course, was simply heavenly, or so some would state. In addition to the sweet and friendly drivers, who 95 percent of the time, engaged in friendly and wholesome conversations with their passengers, riding in a clean, safe, and noiseless vehicle.

The driver's promptness to picking up and arriving to specific destinations was simply impeccable. No one ever complained about long wait times, rude and senseless drivers, and or being dropped off at the wrong locations. In addition, no one complained about arriving to their specific destinations either too early and or way too late. In most passengers' opinion, paratransit was simply as these modern-day people would say, "The bomb!"

Megan, on the other hand, wondered what apparently strong hallucinogenic these people were using to feel this way about the paratransit services. They were clearly fully loaded with some type of illegal substance that blocked every single last one of the common-sense signals that lead straight to their brains. Whatever it was, Megan sometimes whished that she could be given a lifetime prescription of that "good stuff" to make her see through the same rose-colored glasses the other passengers were looking through.

It must be nice to run through the same field of lilies these somewhat distorted people were happily running around in, singing made up little paratransit ditties about how great and wonderful everything was concerning paratransit—its services, vehicles, and especially its drivers.

However, Megan clearly knew that this was not an option to join the crazed few because she dreaded taking any type of medication, and to take something a little extra, in spite of the happy side effects, was a huge no. Besides that, she knew better and had better senses when it came down to the world of paratransit.

While Megan impatiently waited for the paratransit van to show up, she sat sipping on her drink she purchased at the Subway restaurant located inside the West Riverside Walmart. The van was well over an hour late, picking her up from the store. She had placed a call into the paratransit office, inquiring where her van was, and she was told by one of the operators that it would be there in five minutes.

However, that five minutes was sixty minutes ago. In an effort to distract herself and not to become further upset at the late van, Megan mentally started going over her purchases she had made while shopping at the Walmart store. The mental mind-blocking exercise was working until the evil thought popped into her mind about "*him.*"

Megan immediately tried to refocus her thoughts and began to pray silently that *him* would not be the driver to pick her up. She had been pretty blessed for the past few weeks when she had to travel using the paratransit services by not running into *him*, but somehow, Megan feared that today would be the exception.

As her fear of running into *him* increased, beads of perspiration started to form around the edges of her face. Her mouth became immediately dry, and the palms of her hands began to feel sticky and clammy. Her body began bouncing from being extremely hot to severely frigid cold.

"Girl, get yourself together," she said to herself.

"He is not the devil! Although," she continued, "he is not too far from it! Greater is he that lives in me than he that drives that paratransit bus!"

As Megan sat there at the table in the Subway restaurant, mentally focusing on trying to calm herself down, she heard her cell phone ringing. She fished around inside her purse until she came across her phone. Upon retrieving the phone, Megan looked down at the screen and did not recognize the number.

Usually, Megan avoided answering numbers that were not familiar to her because of the increasing number of telemarketers that somehow got a hold of her number, bugging her to try this, buy that, and subscribe to this. But this time around, she was led to answer the call.

"Hello," Megan said.

"Hello, this is Paratransit. I am outside waiting for you," a woman's voice said in response.

Hallelujah! Megan inwardly shouted. It was a female driver picking her up from Walmart and not the dreaded *him*.

As Megan gathered her things together to head out toward the van, she began quietly and happily humming to herself. She had dodged the awful bullet of seeing *him* once again and considered herself to be immensely blessed. More importantly, her body had corrected and regulated itself, and she was no longer in panic mode which was a blessing in itself.

Upon walking through the automatic sliding doors, she saw the paratransit van idling outside with its doors open.

"Hi," the female driver's voice boomed out and continued with sincerity in her voice, "my name is Pamela. I apologize for running behind schedule."

"Oh, it's okay," Megan happily said, smiling up at the driver as she climbed the few steps to get on the bus.

"I don't ever believe I have ever seen you before," Megan said handing the driver her three dollars.

"You are probably right," Pamela said, "I'm a new driver only having started about a month ago."

"Well, welcome to paratransit!" Megan happily said.

"Oh, how sweet of you, and thank you, ma'am," Pamela said, taking Megan's money.

As Megan turned to walk toward the seats, she saw a dark skulking figure of a man grinning at her from the back of the bus. She froze in her steps for a brief moment upon noticing and recognizing that the large, intrusive figure was her nightmare in real life.

It was *him*. The paratransit driver she dreaded seeing.

"Hi, Ms. Sims," the dark looming figured bellowed out, "it is so good seeing you again. I haven't seen you in months. Where in the world have you been hiding?"

Megan woefully sat in the seat farthest from *him* and quietly answered, "I haven't been hiding, only praying."

"What?" The driver exclaimed.

"Never mind," Megan said as she buckled herself in and then arranged her shopping bags on the seat beside her.

"It is my turn to train Pamela today," he stated without anyone's encouragement to speak.

As Pamela pulled off and maneuvered around the Walmart parking lot, edging toward the exit to the main street, a single tear fell from Megan's eye as the dreaded *him* droned on without ceasing.

Readers' note: I have left the full details about the driver, *Him,* a complete and total mystery. Why, you may ask? Well, this is my reasoning. I am giving you the opportunity to plug in your own personal *Him* and/or *Her*, for you to share in the feelings of the main character, Megan.

We all have that one person and/or persons who have rubbed us the wrong way, and it would serve us greatly if we never ran into the person and/or persons again. However, life usually doesn't afford us the opportunity of not seeing a person we dislike and/or not care about unless drastic measures are met.

Seeing that Rockford is truly not a big city at all, we are bound to run into our own dreaded *him* and/or *her* on occasion. It is up to us to determine how we handle that situation. I encourage you to pray and get the victory. If you don't, however, each time you see that particular person, more coals will be added to the fire. The hold that you have given someone over your happiness is clearly not worth it. Please do not be like Megan where you go into a panic attack simply by the mere thought of a person. So let it go and let God and be blessed!

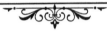

About the Author

Sara Rockford, which is the author's pen name, grew up in Chicago, Illinois, where she obtained a degree in business administration as well as an associate degree in graphic design through Robert Morris University. After relocating to Rockford, Illinois, in 2003, she was diagnosed with having vascular retinopathy in 2005, which is described as a damage to the retina caused by abnormal blood flow.

Due to her newly acquired disability, Sara became a frequent rider of the paratransit division of the Rockford Mass Transit District in 2005. Sara enjoys spending time with other visually impaired individuals through Rockford's Center for Sight and Hearing. Ms. Rockford is also an entrepreneur and business owner. She started her own graphic design business, Touch from Heaven Designs, in 2016 where she designs custom work using various media platforms. *Para-What?* is her first written work.

CPSIA information can be obtained
at www.ICGtesting.com
Printed in the USA
LVHW030536010322
712297LV00001B/132